Copycat]

CW00458501

Tasty Dishes from the Most Famous Restaurants to Make at Home. Cracker Barrel, Red Lobster, Chipotle, Olive Garden, Texas Roadhouse, Applebee's and More.

Gilda Collins

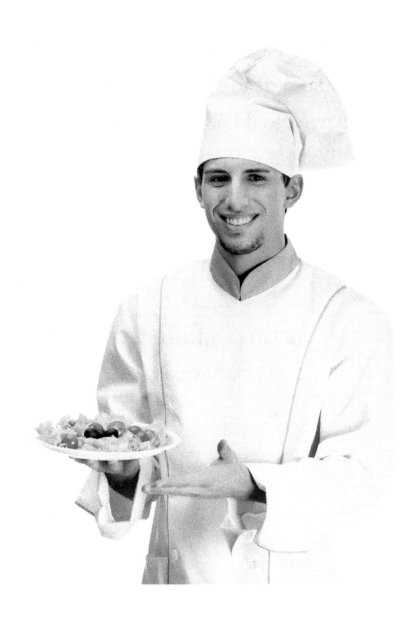

TABLE OF CONTENTS

INTRODUCTION

Copycat Recipes are those recipes that had been adapted from other recipes, generally with a change or two. The original recipe may come from an existing cookbook, noted chef, or even a personal friend.

The popularity of copycat recipes is on the rise. It has been proven that consumers like to try out the latest trend they saw someone else make on television or that their friend served them at a dinner party. More and more people are getting into cooking, more so with the emergence of reality cooking shows where anyone can have the potential of being discovered for having a talent in the kitchen. There are also many cooking shows, both television and online, that feature star-chefs that help people create tasty dishes. Copycat recipes seem to be an easy way out because they require no culinary skills or talent.

Copycat recipes have come a long way since the days where they were limited to a few basic ingredients or simple substitutes for ingredients that was hard to find at supermarkets. Today, some copycat recipes are so elaborate and challenging that the ability to perform an accurate calculation of a recipe is critical if you want it to turn out well.

Copycat recipes have been around for ages. In Los Angeles, where there is a large Mexican-American population, Mexican foods such as fajitas and burritos have become so popular that they are now commonly served at restaurants and fast-food establishments. The popularity of these foods in the United States can be attributed to the fact that a person can order them off menus at restaurants in Mexico or other Latin American countries without having to speak Spanish. Another reason for the popularity of copycat recipes comes from both television and internet exposure where there are recipes that claim to be authentic at least based on a relative chef's recollection while also being easy to prepare. Copycat recipes are considered a cheaper alternative to buying the authentic dish from a restaurant.

People have adapted this style of cooking into a hobby or even a profession. These culinary artists prepare dishes that imitate food served by famous chefs and restaurants such as Gordon Ramsay, Mario Batali, and Paula Deen. These copycat recipes have become so popular that some have been written down in cookbooks for purchase or they can be found online on forums and blogs where they are discussed and shared with other cooks. Most copycat recipes can be found on recipe websites such as those belonging to the Food Network, Allrecipes, Epicurious, and MyRecipes.

Some recipes are considered one-of-a-kind as they come from an individual's kitchen or family history. These are the recipes or variations of them that people have adapted to fit their taste. For example, a family recipe for a well-liked pie might be altered by adding more sugar or less salt. Other times, something new like a combination of pies together is produced in the kitchen through the effort of combining ingredients and flavors for a spectacular and unique final product.

In cooking, some items are not easily found in supermarkets such as fresh herbs and certain meats that may not be popular in one area but could be another part of the country.

So, let us begin?

BREAKFAST RECIPES

IHOP's Buttermilk Pancake

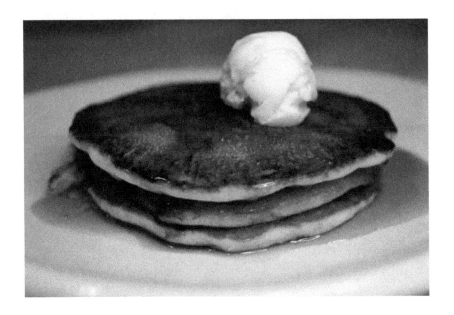

Preparation Time: 5 Minutes

Cooking Time: 8 Minutes

Servings: 8

Ingredients:

- 1¼ cups all-purpose flour
- 1 teaspoon baking soda

- 1 teaspoon baking powder
- 1¼ cups granulated sugar
- 1 pinch salt
- 1 egg
- 1¼ cups buttermilk
- ¼ cup cooking oil

Directions:

1. Preheat your pan by leaving it over medium heat while you are preparing the pancake batter. Incorporate all the dry ingredients together, then combine all of your wet ingredients together as well.

2. Carefully combine the dry mixture into the wet mixture until everything is mixed together completely. Melt some butter in your pan.

3. Slowly pour batter into the pan until you have a 5-inch circle. Flip the pancake when its edges seem to have hardened. Cook the other side of the hotcake as well. Repeat steps six through eight until your batter is finished. Serve with softened butter and maple syrup.

Nutrition: 180 Calories 7.9g Total Fat 23.2g Carbohydrates 4.1g Protein

Starbucks's Marble Pound Cake

Preparation Time: 10 Minutes

Cooking Time: 1 Hour 30 Minutes

Servings: 16

Ingredients:

- 4½ cups cake flour
- 2 teaspoons baking powder
- 1/8 Teaspoon salt
- 6 ounces semisweet chocolate, finely chopped
- 2 cups unsalted butter, softened
- 3 cups granulated sugar
- 1 tablespoon vanilla
- 1 lemon, grated for zest
- 10 large eggs
- 2 tablespoons orange liquor OR milk

Directions:

1. Assemble your ingredients, and then: Preheat the oven to 350F; Grease a 10×4-inch tube pan;

2. Line the pan's bottom with greased wax paper, and Flour the entire pan. Sift together the cake flour, baking powder, and salt in a medium-sized bowl—this is your dry mixture.

3. Melt the chocolate in a medium-sized bowl, then beat in the butter. When it is smooth, mix in the sugar, lemon zest, and vanilla until the liquid mixture is uniform.

4. Beat eggs two at a time, until the mixture looks curdled.

5. Pour half of your dry mixture into your liquid mixture and mix until blended.

6. Add the orange liquor and the rest of the dry mixture. Continue beating the mixture.

7. When the mixture is blended, use a spatula to start folding it—this is your batter.

8. Set aside 4 cups of the batter. Whisk the softened chocolate with the batter.

9. Now that you have a light batter and a dark batter, place the batter into the tube pan by the spoonful, alternating between the two colors.

10.   When the pan is full, shake it slightly to level the batter. Run a knife through the batter to marble it.

11.   Put the dish within the stove and heat for an hour and 15 minutes. In case there are still a

---

few damp pieces on the toothpick after you take it out, at that point, the cake is ready.

12.   Remove the cake and leave it to rest overnight.

Nutrition: 582 Calories 32g Total Fat 69g Carbohydrates 8.6g Protein

IHOP's Scrambled Egg

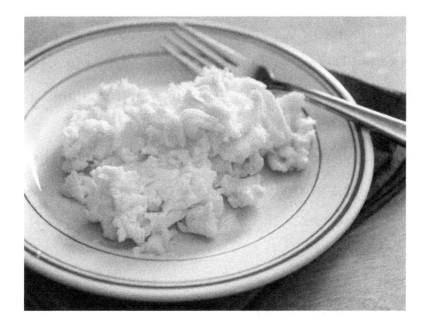

Preparation Time: 5 Minutes

Cooking Time: 5 Minutes

Servings: 1

Ingredients:

- ¼ cup pancake mix
- 1–2 tablespoons butter
- 6 large eggs
- Salt and pepper, to taste

Directions:

1. Thoroughly beat the pancake mix and the eggs together until no lumps or clumps remain.
2. Butter a pan over medium heat. Add in the egg mixture in the middle of the pan. Add the salt and pepper and let the mixture sit for about a minute.
3. When the egg starts cooking, start pushing the edges of the mixture toward the middle of the pan. Continue until the entire mixture is cooked. Serve and enjoy.

Nutrition: 870 Calories 54g Total Fat 9g Carbohydrates 69g Protein

Starbucks's Chocolate Cinnamon Bread

Preparation Time: 15 Minutes

Cooking Time: 60 Minutes

Servings: 16

Ingredients:

Bread:

- 1½ cups unsalted butter
- 3 cups granulated sugar
- 5 large eggs
- 2 cups flour
- 1¼ cups processed cocoa
- 1 tablespoon ground cinnamon
- 1 teaspoon salt
- ½ teaspoon baking powder
- ½ teaspoon baking soda
- ¼ cup water
- 1 cup buttermilk
- 1 teaspoon vanilla extract

Topping:

- ¼ cup granulated sugar
- ½ teaspoon cinnamon

- ½ teaspoon processed cocoa
- 1/8 Teaspoon ginger, ground
- 1/8 Teaspoon cloves, ground

Directions:

1. Grease and preheat the oven to 350 degrees and line the bottoms of the pans with wax paper.

2. Cream the sugar by beating it with the butter. Beat the eggs into the mixture one at a time. Sift the flour, cocoa, cinnamon, salt, baking powder, and baking soda into a large bowl.

3. In another bowl, whisk together the water, buttermilk, and vanilla. Make a well in the dry mixture and start pouring in the wet mixtures a little at a time, while whisking.

4. When the mixture starts becoming doughy, divide it in two, and transfer it to the pans.

5. Combine together all the topping and sprinkle evenly on top of the mixture in both pans.

6. Bake until the bread has set.

Nutrition: 370 Calories 14g Total Fat 59g Carbohydrates 7g Protein

Waffle House's Waffle

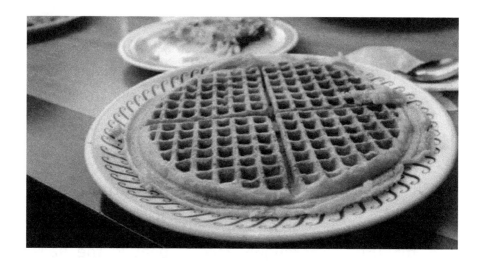

Preparation Time: 5 Minutes

Cooking Time: 20 Minutes

Servings: 6

Ingredients:

- 1½ cups all-purpose flour
- 1 teaspoon salt
- ½ teaspoon baking soda
- 1 egg
- ½ cup + 1 tablespoon granulated white sugar
- 2 tablespoons butter, softened
- 2 tablespoons shortening
- ½ cup half-and-half

- ½ cup milk
- ¼ cup buttermilk
- ¼ teaspoon vanilla

Directions:

1. Prepare the dry mixture by sifting the flour into a bowl and mixing it with the salt and baking soda.

2. Lightly beat an egg until it becomes frothy, beat in the butter, sugar, and shortening. When the mixture is thoroughly mixed, beat in the half-and-half, vanilla, milk, and buttermilk. Continue beating the combination until it is smooth.

3. While beating the wet mixture, slowly pour in the dry mixture, making sure to mix thoroughly and remove all the lumps.

4. Chill the batter overnight (optional but recommended; if you can't chill the mixture overnight, leave it for at least 15 to 20 minutes).

5. Take the batter out of the refrigerator. Preheat and grease your waffle iron.

6. Cook each waffle for three to four minutes. Serve with butter and syrup.

Nutrition: 313 Calories 12g Total Fat 45g Carbohydrates 5.9g Protein

Mimi's Café Santa Fé Omelet

Preparation Time: 10 Minutes

Cooking Time: 10 Minutes

Servings: 1

Ingredients:

Chipotle Sauce:

- 1 cup marinara or tomato sauce
- ¾ cup water
- ½ cup chipotle in adobo sauce
- 1 teaspoon kosher salt

Omelet:

- 1 tablespoon onions, diced
- 1 tablespoon jalapeños, diced
- 2 tablespoons cilantro, chopped
- 2 tablespoons tomatoes, diced
- ¼ cup fried corn tortillas, cut into strips
- 3 eggs, beaten
- 2 slices cheese
- 1 dash of salt and pepper

Garnish:

- 2 ounces chipotle sauce, hot
- ¼ cup fried corn tortillas, cut into strips

- 1 tablespoon sliced green onions
- 1 tablespoon guacamole

Directions:

1. Cook butter over medium heat, making sure to coat the entire pan. Sauté the jalapeños, cilantro, tomatoes, onions, and tortilla strips for about a minute.
2. Pour the eggs, seasoning them with salt and pepper and stirring occasionally. Flip the omelet when it has set. Place the cheese on the top half.
3. When the cheese starts to become melty, fold the omelet in half and transfer to a plate. Garnish the omelet with chipotle sauce, guacamole, green onions, and corn tortillas.

Nutrition: 519 Calories 32g Total Fat 60g Carbohydrates 14g Protein

Alice Springs Chicken from Outback

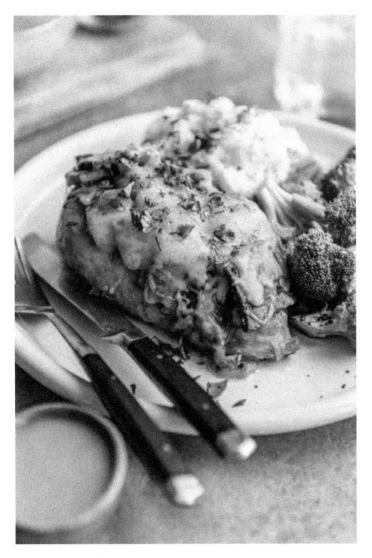

Preparation Time: 5 Minutes

Cooking Time: 2 Hours 30 Minutes

Servings: 4

Ingredients:

Sauce:

- ½ cup Dijon mustard
- ½ cup honey
- ¼ cup mayonnaise
- 1 teaspoon fresh lemon juice

Chicken preparation:

- 4 chicken breast, boneless and skinless
- 2 tablespoons butter
- 1 tablespoon olive oil
- 8 ounces fresh mushrooms, sliced
- 4 slices bacon, cooked and cut into 2-inch pieces
- 2 ½ cups Monterrey Jack cheese, shredded
- Parsley for serving (optional)

Directions:

1. Preheat oven to 400 °F. Mix fixings for the sauce in a bowl.
2. Put the chicken in a Ziploc bag, then add the sauce into the bag until only ¼ cup is left. Keep the remaining sauce in a container, cover, and refrigerate. Make sure to seal the Ziploc bag tightly and shake gently until chicken is coated with sauce. Let it chill for 2 hours.

3. Cook butter in a pan over medium heat. Toss in mushrooms and cook for 5 minutes or until brown. Set aside, then transfer on a plate.

4. In an oven-safe pan, heat oil. Place marinated chicken flat in the pan and cook for 5 minutes on each side or until both sides turn golden brown.

5. Top with even amounts of mushroom, bacon, and cheese. Cover pan with oven-safe lid, then bake for 10 to 15 minutes until chicken is cooked through. Remove lid and bake an additional 1-3 minutes until the cheese is all melted.

6. Transfer onto a plate. Serve with remaining sauce on the side. Sprinkle chicken with parsley if desired

Nutrition: 888 Calories 56g Total Fat 41g Carbohydrates 59g Protein

Oriental Salad from Applebee's

Preparation Time: 15 Minutes

Cooking Time: 5 Minutes

Servings: 6

Ingredients:

- 3 tablespoons honey
- 1½ tablespoons rice wine vinegar
- ¼ cup mayonnaise
- 1 teaspoon Dijon mustard
- 1/8 teaspoon sesame oil
- 3 cups vegetable oil, for frying
- 2 chicken breasts, cut into thin strips
- 1 egg
- 1 cup milk
- 1 cup flour
- 1 cup breadcrumbs
- 1 teaspoon salt
- ¼ teaspoon pepper
- 3 cups romaine lettuce, diced
- ½ cup red cabbage, diced
- ½ cup Napa cabbage, diced
- 1 carrot, grated

- ¼ cup cucumber, diced
- 3 tablespoons sliced almonds
- ¼ cup dry Chow Mein

Directions:

1. To make the dressing, add honey, rice wine vinegar, mayonnaise, Dijon mustard, and sesame oil to a blender. Mix until well combined. Store in refrigerator until ready to serve.

2. Cook oil over medium-high heat in a pan.

3. As the oil warms, whisk together egg and milk in a bowl. In another bowl, add flour, breadcrumbs, salt, and pepper. Mix well.

4. Dredge chicken strips in egg mixture, then in the flour mixture. Make sure the chicken is coated evenly on all sides. Shake off any excess.

5. Deep fry chicken strips for about 3 to 4 minutes until thoroughly cooked and lightly brown. Place onto a plate lined by paper towels to drain and cool. Work in batches, if necessary.

6. Chop strips into small bite-sized pieces once cool enough to handle.

7. Next, prepare the salad by adding romaine, red cabbage, Napa cabbage, carrots, and cucumber

to a serving bowl. Top with chicken pieces, almonds, and chow Mein. Drizzle prepared dressing on top.

8. Serve immediately.

Nutrition: 384 Calories 13g Total Fat 40g Carbohydrates 13g Sugar

Bacon Muffins

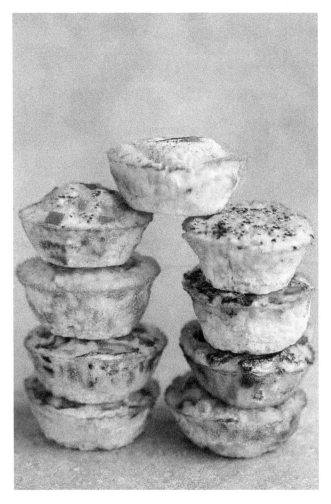

Preparation Time: 5 Minutes

Cooking Time: 15 Minutes

Servings: 4

Ingredients:

- 12.7oz flour
- Salt Pepper

- Egg
- 1 tsp parsley
- Four bacon pieces
- 7.8fl oz milk
- Onion
- 2 tablespoons olive oil
- 3.5ounce Cheddar cheese
- 2 tsp powder

Directions:

1. Preheat oven to 190C/170C fan forced. Line a 12-hole, 1/3 cup–capacity muffin pans with paper cases.
2. Heat oil over medium-high heat. Add bacon. Cook for 5 minutes or until crisp. Cool.
3. Combine sifted flour with pepper, cheese, chives, and bacon in a medium bowl. Make a well in the center. Add remaining ingredients, stirring until combined.
4. Spoon mixture into paper cases. Bake until golden and firm. Stand in pan for 5 minutes. Transfer to wire rack to cool.

Nutrition: 350 Calories 18g Fat 32g Carbohydrates 16g Protein

Breakfast Muffins

Preparation Time: 20 Minutes

Cooking Time: 20 Minutes

Servings: 2

Ingredients:

- New Thyme 1.49fl oz almond milk
- Handfuls lettuce cooked veggies
- Salt Pepper
- 1 tbsp. coriander
- 3oz granola

Directions:

1. Line and preheat the oven at 375 degrees. Transfer and whisk the eggs in a bowl until smooth.
2. Stir in the spinach, bacon, and cheese to the egg mixture to combine. Split the egg mixture evenly among the muffin cups. Bake until eggs are set.
3. Serve immediately. Garnish with diced tomatoes and parsley if desired.

Nutrition: 440 calories 28g Fat 28g Carbohydrates 19g Protein

MAIN RECIPES

Fresh Grilled Salmon

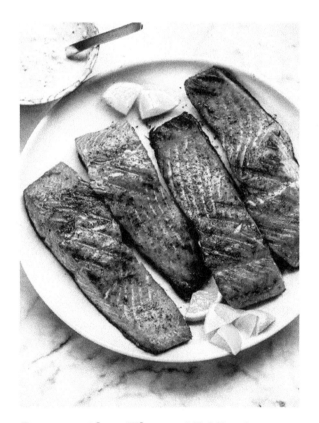

Preparation Time: 15 Minutes

Cooking Time: 10 Minutes

Servings: 6

Ingredients:

- 1/3 cup olive oil
- 3 tablespoons low-sodium soy sauce
- 2 tablespoons Dijon mustard
- ½ teaspoon dried minced garlic
- 6 (5-ounce) salmon fillets

Directions:

1. In a small bowl, add the oil, soy sauce, mustard and garlic and mix well.
2. In a large resealable plastic bag, place half of marinade and salmon fillets.
3. Seal the bag and shake to coat.
4. Refrigerate to marinate for about 30 minutes.
5. Reserve the remaining marinade.
6. Preheat the grill to medium-low heat. Grease the grill grate.
7. Remove the salmon fillets from bag and discard the marinade.
8. Place the salmon fillets onto the grill and cook, covered for about 5-10 minutes or until desired doneness.
9. Transfer the salmon fillets onto a platter and drizzle with reserved marinade.

10.   Serve immediately.

Nutrition: Calories: 290; Total Fat: 20.2g; Saturated Fat: 2.9g Protein: 28.2g; Carbs: 0.9g; Fiber: 0.2g; Sugar: 0.5g

Herb Crusted Salmon

Preparation Time: 15 Minutes

Cooking Time: 13 Minutes

Servings: 4

Ingredients:

- ¾ teaspoon lemon pepper seasoning
- 1 teaspoon dried thyme
- 1 teaspoon dried parsley
- 4 (5-ounce) salmon fillets
- 5 tablespoons fresh lemon juice, divided
- 10 tablespoons butter, divided
- 1 shallot, minced
- 5 tablespoons white wine, divided
- 1 tablespoon white wine vinegar
- 1 cup half-and-half
- Salt and ground white pepper, as required

Directions:

1. In a small bowl, mix together the lemon pepper seasoning and dried herbs.
2. In a shallow dish, place the salmon filets and rub with 3 tablespoons of lemon juice.

3. Season the non-skin side with herb mixture. Set aside.

4. In a sauté pan, melt 2 tablespoons of butter over medium heat.

5. Sauté the shallot for about 2 minutes.

6. Stir in the remaining lemon juice, ¼ cup of wine and vinegar and simmer for about 2-3 minutes.

7. Stir in half-and-half, salt and white pepper and cook for about 2-3 minutes.

8. Add 4 tablespoons of butter and beat until well combined.

9. Remove from the heat and set aside, covered to keep warm.

10. In a wok, melt remaining butter over medium heat.

11. Place salmon in the skillet, herb side down and cook for about 1-2 minutes.

12. Transfer the salmon fillets onto a plate, herb side up.

13. In the wok, add the remaining wine, scraping up the browned bits from bottom.

14. Place the salmon fillets into the wok, herb side up and cook for about 8 minutes.

15.   Transfer the salmon fillets onto serving plates.

16.   Top with pan sauce and serve.

Nutrition: Calories: 547;Total Fat: 44.7g; Saturated Fat: 24g Protein: 29.9g; Carbs: 4.8g; Fiber: 0.3g; Sugar: 0.7g

Southern Fried Catfish

Preparation Time: 15 Minutes

Cooking Time: 4 Minutes

Servings: 4

Ingredients:

- 2 eggs
- 2 tablespoons carbonated water
- 1 cup pancake mix
- ½ teaspoon seasoned salt
- ¼ teaspoon ground black pepper
- 4 (6-ounce) catfish fillets
- 1-2 cups canola oil

Directions:

1. In a shallow bowl, add eggs and water and beat well.
2. In a separate shallow bowl, add the pancake mix, seasoned salt and pepper and mix.
3. Dip the fish fillets in egg mixture, and then coat with seasoned pancake mixture.
4. In a deep skillet, heat the oil over medium-high heat and fry the fish fillets for about 3-4 minutes or until golden brown from both sides.

5. With a slotted spoon, transfer the fish fillets onto a paper towels-lined plate to drain.

6. Serve hot.

Nutrition: Calories: 856; Total Fat: 71.9g; Saturated Fat: 7.4g Protein: 35.2g; Carbs: 17.5g; Fiber: 7.5g; Sugar: 0.2g

Fish & Chips

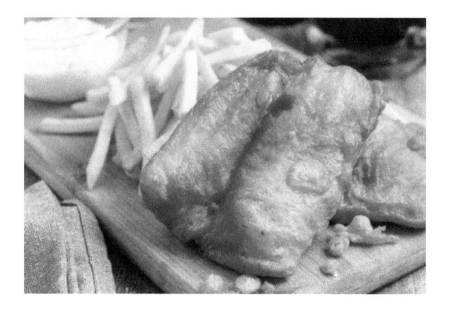

Preparation Time: 15 Minutes

Cooking Time: 20 Minutes

Servings: 4

Ingredients:

- 4 cups frozen steak fries
- 4 (6-ounce) salmon fillets
- 1-2 tablespoons prepared horseradish
- 1 tablespoon Parmesan cheese, grated
- 1 tablespoon Worcestershire sauce
- 1 teaspoon Dijon mustard

- Salt, to taste
- ½ cup panko breadcrumbs
- Cooking spray

Directions:

1. Preheat the oven to 450 degrees F. Arrange a rack in the lower portion of oven. Arrange a second rack in the middle portion of oven.
2. Arrange steak fries onto a baking sheet in a single layer.
3. Place the baking sheet of steak fries onto the lower rack and bake for about 18-20 minutes or until light golden brown.
4. Meanwhile, place salmon on a foil-lined baking sheet coated with cooking spray.
5. In a small bowl, add the horseradish, cheese, Worcestershire sauce, mustard, salt and mix well. Stir in the panko.
6. Coat the salmon fillets with cheese mixture and spray with cooking spray.
7. Arrange the salmon fillets onto a greased baking dish in a single layer.

8. Arrange the baking dish over the middle rack and bake for about 8-10 minutes. or until fish just begins to flake easily with a fork.

9. Serve cod fillets with fries.

Nutrition: Calories: 41; Total Fat: 16.8g; Saturated Fat: 2g Protein: 36g; Carbs: 23.3g; Fiber: 3.2g; Sugar: 2.1g

Fish Taco

Preparation Time: 15 Minutes

Cooking Time: 8 Minutes

Servings: 4

Ingredients:

- ½ cup mayonnaise
- 1 tablespoon fresh lime juice
- 2 teaspoons milk
- 1 large egg
- 1 teaspoon water
- 1/3 cup dry breadcrumbs
- 2 tablespoons lemon-pepper seasoning
- 1 pound cod fillets, cut into 1-inch strips
- 4 (6-inch) corn tortillas, warmed

- 1 cup coleslaw mix
- 2 medium tomatoes, chopped

- 1 cup Mexican cheese blend, shredded

- 1 tablespoon fresh cilantro, minced

Directions:

1. For sauce, in a small bowl, add the mayonnaise, lime juice and milk and mix well.
2. Refrigerate the sauce until serving.
3. In a shallow bowl, add the egg and water and beat well.
4. In another shallow bowl, add the breadcrumbs and lemon pepper seasoning and mix.
5. Dip the cod strips in egg mixture and then coat with breadcrumb mixture.
6. Heat a large nonstick skillet over medium-high heat and cook the cod strips for about 2-4 minutes per side or until golden brown.
7. Arrange the tortillas onto serving plates.
8. Divide cod strips onto each tortilla and top with coleslaw mix, tomatoes, cheese blend and cilantro.
9. Serve alongside the sauce.

Nutrition: Calories: 365; Total Fat: 23.3g; Saturated Fat: 8.2g Protein: 32g; Carbs: 33.7g; Fiber: 4g; Sugar: 4.5g

Bristo Shrimp Pasta

Preparation Time: 15 Minutes

Cooking Time: 10 Minutes

Servings: 2

Ingredients:

- 4 ounces uncooked angel hair pasta
- ¼ cup olive oil
- 8 jumbo shrimp, peeled and deveined
- 6 fresh asparagus spears, trimmed and cut into 2-inch pieces
- 2 garlic cloves, minced
- ½ cup fresh mushrooms, sliced
- 1 small plum tomato, peeled, seeded and chopped
- Salt, to taste
- ½ cup chicken broth
- 1/8 teaspoon red pepper flakes, crushed
- 1 tablespoon fresh basil, minced

- 1 tablespoon oregano, minced
- 1 tablespoon thyme, minced
- 1 tablespoon parsley, minced
- ¼ cup Parmesan cheese, grated

Directions:

1. In a large pan of lightly salted boiling water, cook the pasta for about 8-10 minutes or until according to package's directions.
2. Drain the pasta completely.
3. Meanwhile, in a large wok, heat the oil over medium heat and cook the shrimp and asparagus for about 3-4 minutes.
4. Add the garlic and cook for about 1 minute.
5. Add the mushrooms, tomato, pepper flakes and broth and simmer for about 2 minutes.
6. Add the pasta and herbs and toss to coat.
7. Serve hot with the sprinkling of cheese

Nutrition: Calories: 572; Total Fat: 31.4g; Saturated Fat: 5.7g Protein: 34.9g; Carbs: 41.3g; Fiber: 3.9g; Sugar: 3.2g

Shrimp Scampi

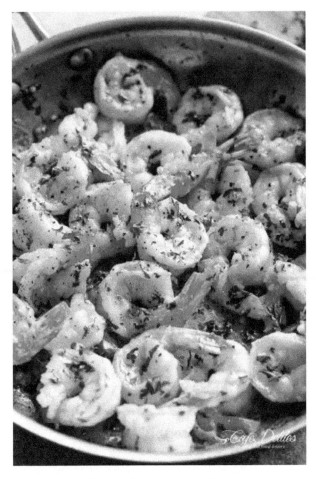

Preparation Time: 20 Minutes

Cooking Time: 55 Minutes

Servings: 6

Ingredients:

- 1 cup milk

- 4 tablespoons parmesan cheese, grated finely and divided
- ½ cup all-purpose flour
- ¼ teaspoon cayenne pepper
- Salt and ground black pepper, as required
- 2 pounds shrimp, peeled, deveined and butterflied
- 2 cups olive oil
- 6-8 whole garlic cloves, peeled
- 1 cup dry white wine
- 2 cups heavy cream
- 1 tomato, chopped
- 1 shallot, chopped
- 5 -7 fresh basil leaves, shredded
- 1 pound angel hair pasta
- 3 tablespoons fresh parsley, chopped

Directions:

1. In a large shallow bowl, place the milk.
2. In a separate shallow bowl, add flour, 2 tablespoons of cheese, cayenne pepper, salt and black pepper and mix well.
3. Dip the shrimp in milk and then coat with flour mixture.

4. In a deep skillet, heat the oil over medium-high heat and fry the shrimp in 3 batches for about 2 minutes per sides.

5. With a slotted spoon, transfer the fish shrimp onto a paper towels-lined plate to drain.

6. With a paper towel, cover the shrimp to keep them warm.

7. In a wok, heat 2 tablespoons of oil and over medium-low heat and sauté the garlic for about 1-2 minutes.

8. Add the wine and bring it to a boil.

9. Adjust the heat to low and simmer, covered for about 10-15 minutes.

10. Add the cream and bring a boil.

11. Adjust the heat to low and simmer for about 10 more minutes.

12. Add the tomato, shallots, basil and remaining Parmesan cheese and cook for about 1 minute, stirring frequently.

13. Stir in the fried shrimp and remove from the heat.

14. Set aside to cool slightly.

---

15. In a large pan of lightly salted boiling water, cook the pasta for about 8-10 minutes or until according to package's directions.

16. Drain the pasta completely.

17. Divide pasta onto serving plates and top with shrimp sauce.

18. Garnish with parsley and serve immediately.

Nutrition: Calories: 1188; Total Fat: 87.2g; Saturated Fat: 20g Protein: 46g; Carbs: 55.6g; Fiber: 0.6g; Sugar: 2.5g

Cajun Jambalaya Pasta

Preparation Time: 15 Minutes

Cooking Time: 15 Minutes

Servings: 6

Ingredients:

- 1 pound chicken breast, cut into 1-inch pieces
- ½ pound shrimp, peeled and deveined
- ½ pound Andouille sausage, cut into 1-inch-thick pieces
- 3 tablespoons Cajun spice blend
- ½ of red bell pepper, seeded and chopped
- ½ of green bell pepper, seeded and chopped
- ½ of red onion, sliced thinly
- 3 garlic cloves, minced
- Salt and ground black pepper, as required
- 3 tablespoons canola oil
- 1 medium tomato, chopped
- 1 cup chicken broth
- 1-pound cooked fettuccine pasta
- 3 tablespoons fresh parsley, chopped

Directions:

1. In a large bowl add the chicken, shrimp, sausage, Cajun spices, bell peppers, onion, garlic, salt and black pepper and mix well.
2. In a large cast iron skillet, heat the canola oil over high heat.
3. Add the chicken mixture in 2 batches and sear for about 4-5 minutes.
4. In the skillet, add the tomatoes and broth with all the chicken mixture and cook for about 1-2 minutes.
5. Add the cooked pasta and toss to coat well.
6. Garnish with parsley and serve immediately.

Nutrition: Calories: 564; Total Fat: 22g; Saturated Fat: 4.6g Protein: 41.9g; Carbs: 47.5g; Fiber: 0.9g; Sugar: 2.4g

Cobb Salad

Preparation Time: 15 Minutes

Cooking Time: 0 Minutes

Servings: 6

Ingredients:

For Dressing

- ¾cup canola oil
- ¼ cup olive oil
- ¼ cup red wine vinegar
- 1 teaspoon lemon juice
- ¾ teaspoon Worcestershire sauce
- 1 small garlic clove, minced
- ¼ teaspoon sugar
- ¼ teaspoon ground mustard
- Salt and ground black pepper, as required

For Salad:

- 2 cooked chicken breasts, chopped
- 6 cooked bacon strips, crumbled
- 6½ cups romaine lettuce, torn
- 2½ cups curly endive, torn
- 4 ounces watercress, trimmed and divided
- 2 medium tomatoes, seeded and chopped

- 1 medium ripe avocado, peeled, pitted and chopped
- 3 hard-boiled large eggs, peeled and chopped
- ½ cup blue cheese, crumbled
- 2 tablespoons fresh chives, minced

Directions:

1. For dressing: in a blender, add all ingredients and pulse until smooth.
2. Transfer the dressing into a bowl and refrigerate before serving.
3. For salad: in a large salad bowl, add all ingredients and mix.
4. Cover the bowl and refrigerate to chill before serving.
5. Just before serving, drizzle salad with dressing and serve.

Nutrition: Calories: 747; Total Fat: 64.5g; Saturated Fat: 12.6g Protein: 34.7g; Carbs: 8.4g; Fiber: 4g; Sugar: 2.4g

White Chicken Chili

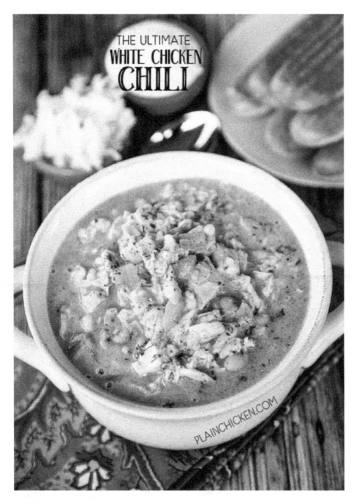

Preparation Time: 15 Minutes

Cooking Time: 25 Minutes

Servings: 6

Ingredients:

- 2 (15-ounce) cans cannellini beans, rinsed and drained

- 1-pound lean ground chicken
- 1 medium onion, chopped
- 1 (4-ounce) can chopped green chiles
- ½ teaspoon dried oregano
- 1 teaspoon ground cumin
- ¼ teaspoon ground black pepper
- 1 (14½-ounces) can low-sodium chicken broth

Directions:

1. In a small bowl, add 1 can of beans and mash slightly. Set aside.
2. Heat a large nonstick saucepan over medium-high heat and cook the chicken and onion for about 6-8 minutes, breaking up chicken into crumbles.
3. Stir in the mashed beans, remaining can of beans, chiles, oregano, cumin, black pepper and broth and bring to a boil.
4. Adjust the heat to low and simmer, covered for about 12-15 minutes.
5. Serve hot.

Nutrition: Calories: 592; Total Fat: 5.3g; Saturated Fat: 1.5g Protein: 49.6g; Carbs: 88.6g; Fiber: 35.8g; Sugar: 4.6g

SNACK RECIPES

Cracker Jack

Preparation Time: 30 Minutes

Cooking Time: 25 Minutes

Servings: 3

Ingredients:

- 4 quarts popcorn, popped
- ½ cup peanuts
- 3 tablespoons butter
- 1/3 cup dark brown sugar
- ½ cup light corn syrup
- 3 tablespoons molasses
- Pinch of salt

Directions:

1. Preheat oven to 275°F.
2. Take a small bowl and add popcorn and peanuts.

3. Place the bowl in the preheated oven for 5 minutes.
4. Meanwhile, take a saucepan and heat butter, sugar, corn syrup, salt, and molasses.
5. Cook for approximately 10 minutes, until mixture boils.
6. Once the mixture boils, turn the stove off.
7. Take out the popcorn and peanuts from the oven.
8. Pour the prepared caramel on top.
9. Reheat in the oven for 10 minutes.
10. Once popcorn and peanuts are coated well take it out.
11. Let cool and then serve.

Nutrition: Calories 669, total fat 25.5 g, carbs 108 g, Protein 11.9 g, sodium 153 mg

Chex Mix Party Blend

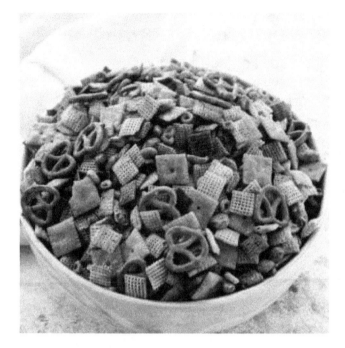

Preparation Time: 15 Minutes

Cooking Time: 5 Minutes

Servings: 4

Ingredients:

- 1 tablespoon margarine
- ½ teaspoon soy sauce
- 2 tablespoons canola oil
- ½ teaspoon onion powder
- 4 teaspoons Worcestershire sauce
- 1½ teaspoons cheddar popcorn seasoning
- ½ teaspoon garlic powder

- 1 cup Corn Chex
- 1 cup Wheat Chex
- 1 cup pretzels
- 2 cups mini-crackers
- 1 cup mini-breadsticks

Directions:

1. Preheat the oven to 340°F.
2. Take a bowl and add margarine to it.
3. Melt margarine in the oven.
4. Add the oil, soy sauce and Worcestershire sauce.
5. Add the garlic powder, popcorn seasoning, and onion powder to the bowl.
6. Mix well.
7. Take a separate bowl and mix the Corn Chex, Wheat Chex, pretzels, mini-crackers and mini-breadsticks.
8. Pour the blended mixture into the cracker mixture.
9. Whisk well.
10. Pour the mixture into the baking dish and bake in the oven for 5 minutes.
11. Once cooled, serve.

Nutrition: Calories 462, total fat 0.3 g, carbs 70.2 g, Protein 8.5 g, sodium 1084 mg

Nabisco Cheese Nips

Preparation Time: 20 Minutes

Cooking Time: 10 Minutes

Servings: 5

Ingredients:

- 1 cup all-purpose flour, sifted (plus ½ cup reserved)
- ½ teaspoon baking soda
- ½ teaspoon baking powder
- 1/3 cup Kraft Macaroni & Cheese topping powder
- ¼ cup shortening
- ½ cup buttermilk
- 1/3 teaspoon salt (for topping)

Directions:

1. Preheat oven to 250°F.
2. Oil a baking sheet and set aside.
3. In a bowl, sift one cup of flour with cheese powder, baking soda, and baking powder.
4. Add the shortening and work with a fork until broken down into rice-size pieces.

5. Mix buttermilk into flour mixture until a moist dough is formed.
6. Sprinkle reserved flour over the dough and work it until it is no longer sticky.
7. Chill the dough for 1 hour.
8. Remove the dough from the refrigerator and start rolling it out while sprinkling reserved flour on top.
9. Roll to 1/6 of an inch thick and then trim the edges.
10. Transfer the dough to the baking sheet.
11. Create 1-inch-square pieces (a pizza cutter would be perfect for this).
12. Make a hole in the center of each piece with a toothpick.
13. Sprinkle salt on top and bake in the oven for 8–10 minutes, until lightly browned.
14. Serve.

Nutrition: Calories 220, total fat 11.8 g, carbs 23.8 g, Protein 3.4 g, sodium 608 mg

Ranch Doritos

Preparation Time: 25 Minutes

Cooking Time: 15 Minutes

Servings: 10

Ingredients:

Seasoning Mix

- ½ cup dry ranch dressing mix
- 3 tablespoons white cheddar cheese powder
- 4 teaspoons paprika
- 4 teaspoons dried tomato powder
- 2 teaspoons garlic, granulated
- 2 teaspoons onion, granulated
- 2 teaspoons of popcorn salt, powdered

Tortilla Wedges

- Corn tortillas, as needed (cut into wedges)
- 1 cup peanut oil, for frying

Directions:

1. Combine all the seasoning mix ingredients in a bowl.
2. Heat oil in a pan.
3. Line a bowl with paper towels.

4. Place an additional large heatproof bowl to the side.

5. Once the oil gets hot, add tortilla wedges and fry till crisp.

6. Put them in the paper towel bowl to begin with.

7. Then transfer to the large heatproof bowl.

8. Sprinkle a few teaspoons of seasoning mix over the wedges and toss to mix well.

9. Repeat the process until all the wedges are done and coated well.

10. Serve after a day.

Nutrition: Calories 259, total fat 22.7 g, carbs 12.2 g, Protein 2.6 g, sodium 245 mg

Corn Dog

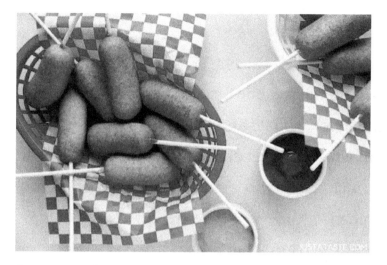

Preparation Time: 10 Minutes

Cooking Time: 5 Minutes

Servings: 20

Ingredients:

- 2 cups yellow cornmeal
- 2 cups all-purpose flour
- ½ teaspoon salt
- ¼ teaspoon black pepper
- 1 cup white sugar
- 2 tablespoons baking powder
- 2 eggs, whisked
- 2 cups milk
- 2 quarts vegetable oil, for frying

- 24 ounces package beef frankfurters

Equipment

- 26–28 wooden skewers

Directions:

1. In a large mixing bowl, combine flour, cornmeal, salt, pepper, sugar, and baking powder.
2. Stir in whisked eggs and mix all ingredients well.
3. Add milk and mix until all ingredients are combined.
4. Preheat the oil in a large pan.
5. Insert the skewers into the frankfurters.
6. Roll frankfurters in the batter.
7. Once coated fully, fry in oil for 3 minutes.
8. Drain excess oil on paper towels.

Nutrition: Calories 1029, total fat 98 g, carbs 32 g, Protein 7.5 g, sodium 470 mg

Old El Paso Refried Beans

Preparation Time: 4 Hours

Cooking Time: 4 Hours

Servings: 8

Ingredients:

- 30 ounces refried beans
- 2 cups onions, diced
- 2 pounds Mexican cheese
- 32 ounce-jar salsas
- 1 cup green onion, chopped
- ½ cup sour cream, or to taste
- 1 cup black olives, or to taste
- 1 cup cherry tomatoes, or to taste

Directions:

1. Add beans, onions, half of cheese and salsa to a crockpot and cook for 3 hours on high.
2. Add the rest of the cheese, green onions, and sliced olives and cook for another hour.
3. Open the pot and add sour cream and tomatoes.
4. Serve.

Nutrition: Calories 606, total fat 41.7 g, carbs 34 g, Protein 30 g, sodium 1681 mg

Sabra Hummus

Preparation Time: 5 Minutes

Cooking Time: 0 Minutes

Servings: 4

Ingredients:

- 1 (14-ounce) can chickpeas, drained
- 1/3 cup tahini sauce
- Juice of 1 lemon
- 2 cloves garlic
- Salt and black pepper, to taste
- 1 teaspoon olive oil

Directions:

1. Use a high-speed blender to blend all the ingredients thoroughly.
2. Serve and enjoy.

Nutrition: Calories 576, total fat 27 g, carbs 65.5 g, Protein 24 g, sodium 205 mg

Rondelé Garlic & Herbs Cheese Spread

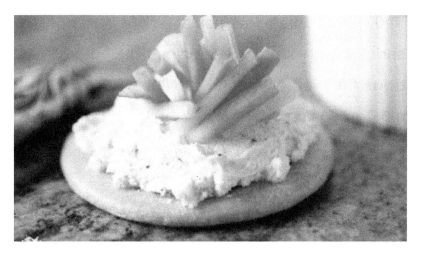

Preparation Time: 5 Minutes

Cooking Time: 0 Minutes

Servings: 4

Ingredients:

- 18 ounces cream cheese, whipped
- 2 teaspoons fresh garlic, finely minced
- 1 teaspoon Italian seasoning
- ½ teaspoon salt
- ¼ teaspoon onion powder
- Sliced green onions for garnish

Directions:

1. Combine all the ingredients in a bowl and then transfer to a glass jar.
2. Refrigerate for a few hours before serving and sprinkle with sliced green onions.

Nutrition: Calories 451, total fat 44 g, carbs 4.1 g, Protein 9.7 g, sodium 669 mg

Lipton Onion Soup Mix

Preparation Time: 5 Minutes

Cooking Time: 0 Minutes

Servings: 2

Ingredients:

- 1½ cups dry onion flakes
- ½ cup beef bouillon powder
- 8 teaspoons onion powder
- ½ teaspoon crushed celery seeds
- ½ teaspoon dry parsley
- ½ teaspoon sugar

Directions:

1. Combine all ingredients in a jar.
2. Store it with an airtight cover.

Nutrition: Calories 19, total fat 0.4 g, carbs 4.2 g, Protein 0.7 g, sodium 192 mg

Progresso Italian Style Bread Crumbs

Preparation Time: 10 Minutes

Cooking Time: 0 Minutes

Servings: 5

Ingredients:

- 4 cups bread crumbs, plain and dry
- 1 teaspoon garlic powder
- ½ teaspoon onion powder
- 1 tablespoon white sugar
- 1 teaspoon kosher salt
- 2 teaspoons parsley, dried
- 1/3 teaspoon oregano, dried

Directions:

1. Mix all the ingredients in a bowl.
2. Store in an airtight container and use as needed.

Nutrition: Calories 353, total fat 0.6 g, carbs 65 g, Protein 12 g, sodium 1098 mg

SOUP, SIDE, AND SALAD RECIPES

Vegetable Soup

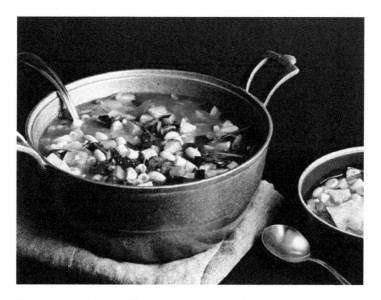

Preparation Time: 10 Minutes

Cooking Time: 60 Minutes

Servings: 5

Ingredients:

- 12 oz frozen peas
- 12 oz frozen corn
- 12 oz frozen lima beans

- 10 oz frozen onions
- 28 oz can tomato, diced
- 16 oz can green beans
- 2 large potatoes, peeled and cubed
- 2 celery stalks, sliced
- 5 cups vegetable stock
- 4 beef bouillon cubes
- 5 cups of water
- 1 tsp ground black pepper
- 1 tsp salt

Directions:

1. Add all ingredients into the large pot and bring to boil.
2. Reduce heat to medium, cover, and cook for 1 hour.
3. Stir well and serve.

Nutrition: Calories: 677; Total Fat: 5.9g; Saturated Fat: 1.4g; Protein: 28.5g; Carbs: 146.5g; Fiber: 32g; Sugar: 32.6g

Cole Slaw

Preparation Time: 10 Minutes

Cooking Time: 10 Minutes

Servings: 8

Ingredients:

- 2 bags coleslaw cabbage mix
- ¼ tsp celery seeds
- 1 tsp vinegar
- 4 tsp fresh lemon juice
- ¼ cup buttermilk
- ¼ cup milk
- ½ cup mayonnaise
- ¼ tsp salt

Directions:

1. Add coleslaw cabbage mix into the large mixing bowl.
2. In a small bowl, mix together mayonnaise, milk, buttermilk, lemon juice, vinegar, celery seeds, and salt and pour over coleslaw and mix well.
3. Place coleslaw into the refrigerator for 2 hours before serving.
4. Serve and enjoy.

Nutrition: Calories: 105; Total Fat: 10g; Saturated Fat: 1g; Protein: 0.9g; Carbs: 5.6g; Fiber: 0.5g; Sugar: 1g

Mashed Potatoes

Preparation Time: 10 Minutes

Cooking Time: 55 Minutes

Servings: 6

Ingredients:

- 6 large potatoes, peeled & cubed
- 1 stick margarine, cut into pieces
- 8 oz can evaporate milk
- Pepper
- Salt

Directions:

1. Add potatoes and salt into the boiling water and cook until tender. Drain potatoes well.
2. Transfer potatoes into the mixing bowl. Add margarine. Slowly add milk and mashed the potatoes using a hand mixer until smooth and creamy.
3. Season with pepper and salt.
4. Serve and enjoy.

Nutrition: Calories: 422; Total Fat: 15.5g; Saturated Fat: 2.6g; Protein: 8.9g; Carbs: 63.2g; Fiber: 8.9g; Sugar: 9.3g

Baby Lima Beans

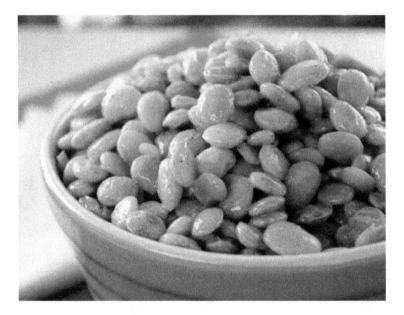

Preparation Time: 10 Minutes

Cooking Time: 60 Minutes

Servings: 8

Ingredients:

- 16 oz frozen baby lima beans
- 1/8 tsp red pepper flakes
- ½ tsp black pepper
- 1 tsp sugar
- ½ tsp onion powder
- 1 garlic clove, minced
- 1 ½ cups chicken stock
- 2 bacon slices, sliced

- Salt

Directions:

1. Add bacon slices into the large pot and sauté for 1-2 minutes.
2. Add remaining ingredients and stir everything well. Cover and bring to boil. Reduce heat and simmer for 30 minutes.
3. Stir well and cook for 30 minutes more or until beans are tender.
4. Serve and enjoy.

Nutrition: Calories: 74;Total Fat: 1g; Saturated Fat: 0.3g; Protein: 4.3g;

Carbs: 12.4g; Fiber: 2.8g; Sugar: 1.5g

Baby Carrots

Preparation Time: 10 Minutes

Cooking Time: 45 Minutes

Servings: 8

Ingredients:

- 2 lbs. fresh baby carrots, rinse
- 1 tbsp brown sugar
- 2 tbsp margarine
- 1 tsp salt

Directions:

1. Add carrots into the large saucepan. Pour enough water to cover the carrots.
2. Cover pan with lid and cook over medium heat. Bring to boil.
3. Reduce heat to low and simmer for 45 minutes or until carrots are tender.
4. Once carrots are tender then drain half of the water from carrots.
5. Add sugar, margarine, and salt to the carrots and stir well. Cover the pan again with lid and cook until carrots are completely tender.
6. Serve and enjoy.

Nutrition: Calories: 69; Total Fat: 3g; Saturated Fat: 0.5g; Protein: 0.8g; Carbs: 10.5g; Fiber: 3.3g; Sugar: 6.5g

Country Style Green Beans

Preparation Time: 10 Minutes

Cooking Time: 50 Minutes

Servings: 6

Ingredients:

- 43.5 oz can whole green beans, do not drain
- 1 tsp sugar
- ½ cup sweet onion, diced
- ¼ lb. bacon, chopped
- ½ tsp black pepper
- ½ tsp salt

Directions:

1. Add onion and bacon in a saucepan and cook over medium-high heat until they begin to brown. Stir frequently.
2. Add green beans, sugar, pepper, and salt and stir everything well.
3. Cover saucepan, turn heat to low, and cook for 45 minutes.
4. Stir well and serve warm.

Nutrition: Calories: 254; Total Fat: 7.9g; Saturated Fat: 2.6g; Protein: 14.4g; Carbs: 31g; Fiber: 14.8g; Sugar: 15.6g

Mac and Cheese

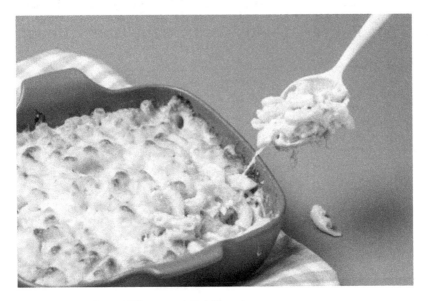

Preparation Time: 10 Minutes

Cooking Time: 30 Minutes

Servings: 6

Ingredients:

- 2 ½ cups pasta, uncooked
- ½ cup parmesan cheese, grated
- ½ cup Velveeta cheese, cut into small cubes
- 2 cups Colby cheese, shredded
- ½ cup cream
- 1 cup chicken broth, low-sodium
- 2 tbsp flour
- 2 tbsp butter

- 1 tsp salt

Directions:

1. Preheat the oven to 350 F/ 180 C. Grease 8*8-inch casserole dish and set aside.
2. Cook pasta according to the packet instructions.
3. Melt butter in a pan over medium heat. Slowly whisk in flour.
4. Whisk constantly and slowly add the broth.
5. Slowly pour the cream and whisk constantly.
6. Slowly add parmesan cheese, Velveeta cheese, and Colby cheese and whisk until it is a smooth sauce.
7. Add cooked pasta to the sauce and stir everything well to coat.
8. Transfer pasta into the prepared casserole dish and bake in preheated oven for 15 minutes.
9. Serve and enjoy.

Nutrition: Calories: 404; Total Fat: 24.2g; Saturated Fat: 15.2g; Protein: 20.9g; Carbs: 22.8g; Fiber: 2g; Sugar: 1.4g

Corn Muffins

Preparation Time: 10 Minutes

Cooking Time: 20 Minutes

Servings: 8

Ingredients:

- 2 eggs
- ½ cup unsalted butter, melted
- ¾ cup buttermilk
- 1 tbsp honey
- ½ cup sugar
- 1 ¼ cups self-rising flour
- ¾ cup yellow cornmeal

Directions:

1. Preheat the oven to 350 F/ 180 C. Line a 12-cup muffin pan with paper liners.
2. In a large bowl, mix together cornmeal, sugar, and flour.
3. In a separate bowl, whisk the eggs with buttermilk and honey until well combined.
4. Slowly add egg mixture and melted butter to the cornmeal mixture and stir until just mixed.

5. Spoon batter into the prepared muffin pan and bake in preheated oven for 18-20 minutes.

6. Remove muffin from oven and let it cool for 5 minutes then serve warm.

Nutrition: Calories: 294; Total Fat: 13.4g; Saturated Fat: 7.9g; Protein: 5.2g; Carbs: 39.6g; Fiber: 1.4g; Sugar: 16g

Fried Apples

Preparation Time: 10 Minutes

Cooking Time: 20 Minutes

Servings: 10

Ingredients:

- 4 medium apples, cored & cut into ¾-inch wedges
- 1 tbsp cornstarch
- ½ cup apple cider
- ¼ tsp ground nutmeg
- 1 tsp ground cinnamon
- 2 tbsp brown sugar
- ¼ cup granulated sugar
- 3 tbsp butter

Directions:

1. Melt butter in a pan over medium heat.
2. Add apples, spices, and sugars and stir to coat. Cover the pan with a lid and cook for 10-15 minutes, stirring occasionally, until tender.
3. Transfer apples to serving dish. Cover and set aside.

4. In a small bowl, whisk together cornstarch and apple cider and add to the same pan. Cook over medium heat, stirring continuously to blend. Simmer for 40-60 seconds or until thickened.

5. Pour cornstarch mixture over apples and mix well.

6. Serve warm and enjoy.

Nutrition: Calories: 112; Total Fat: 3.7g; Saturated Fat: 2.2g; Protein: 0.3g; Carbs: 21.5g; Fiber: 2.3g; Sugar: 17.4g

Fried Okra

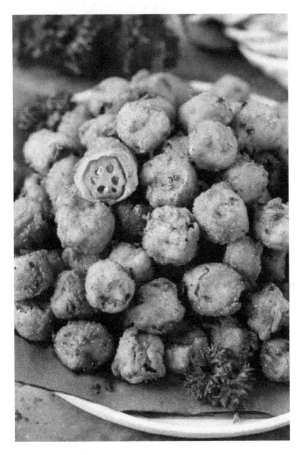

Preparation Time: 10 Minutes

Cooking Time: 15 Minutes

Servings: 2

Ingredients:

- 1 ½ cups okra, sliced
- 1/8 tsp black pepper
- ¼ tsp garlic herb seasoning blend

- 2 tbsp cornmeal
- 2 tbsp all-purpose flour
- 3 tbsp buttermilk
- ¼ tsp salt

Directions:

1. Pat dry sliced okra with a paper towel.
2. In a shallow bowl, add buttermilk.
3. In a separate shallow bowl, mix together flour, seasoning, cornmeal, pepper, and salt.
4. Dip okra in buttermilk then coat with flour mixture.
5. In a deep fat fryer heat 1-inch of oil to 375 F/ 190 C. Fry few pieces of okra at a time for 1-2 minutes on each side or until lightly golden brown.
6. Drain on paper towels. Season with pepper and salt.
7. Serve and enjoy.

Nutrition: Calories: 368; Total Fat: 31g; Saturated Fat: 2g; Protein: 5g;
Carbs: 19g; Fiber: 4g; Sugar: 4g

DESSERT RECIPES

Cinnabon's Monkey Bread

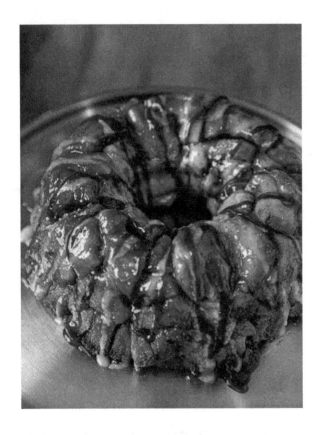

Preparation Time: 5 Minutes

Cooking Time: 20 Minutes

Servings: 4

Ingredients:

- 3 cans Cinnabon cinnamon roll dough
- 1 cup sugar
- 1 tablespoon cinnamon
- ½ cup (1 stick) butter, melted
- ½ cup brown sugar
- 2 tablespoons honey

Frosting

- 1 tablespoon milk
- 1 teaspoon butter
- 2 cups powdered sugar

Directions:

1. Preheat oven to 400°F. Grease a Bundt or loaf pan.
2. Cut each dough roll into half and roll into balls.
3. Combine sugar and cinnamon and place in a plastic bag or shallow dish.
4. Coat the dough with the cinnamon sugar.
5. Fit the dough into the pan.
6. In a bowl, stir the butter, brown sugar and honey together until all the sugar is dissolved.
7. Pour the honey mixture evenly over the dough in the pan.

8. Bake until fragrant and browned, or with internal temperature of 190–200°F (about 20 minutes).

9. If using frosting, prepare it while the bread is baking. Then, place ingredients in a saucepan over low heat; stirring continuously until smooth. It should be a good consistency for drizzling. Add a few drops of water or milk if too thick.

10. Let the bread cool down for about 5 minutes before removing

from the pan. Drizzle with frosting

Nutrition: Calories: 922; Total Fat: 23.9g; Saturated Fat: 10.6g; Protein: 13.1g; Carbs: 165g; Fiber: 4.9g; Sugar: 104.1g

Starbucks Chia Latte Copycat

Preparation Time: 5 Minutes

Cooking Time: 0 Minutes

Servings: 5

Ingredients:

- Ground cardamom, for garnish
- 2 cinnamon sticks
- 1 star anise
- 6 cardamom pods
- 1/3 cup packed brown sugar
- Ground cinnamon, for garnish
- 4 cups whole milk
- 6 black tea bags
- 2 tablespoons whole cloves
- 1 tablespoon black peppercorns
- 1 1-inch piece fresh ginger, thinly sliced
- 4 cups water
- 1 tablespoon vanilla extract, pure

Directions:

1. First, in a small pot, bring the water, sugar and spices to boil over medium heat. You can reduce

the heat and allow them to cook for like 5 minutes.

2. Bring the mixture back to a boil. Add the vanilla and tea bags and remove from heat. Cover for 10 minutes and allow to steep. Then, strain tea bags and discard spices.

3. Next, bring the milk to a simmer in a medium pot over medium heat. Turn off heat and use a froth milk immersion blender.

4. Pour 3/4 cup chai tea and 1/2 cup warm milk into each mug, changing amounts according to preferences. Round off each mug with milk foam and cinnamon and cardamom sprinkled on the top.

Nutrition: Calories: 671; Total Fat: 31.3g; Saturated Fat: 14.6g; Protein: 5.3g; Carbs: 98.4g; Fiber: 2.3g; Sugar: 76.2g

Oriental Salad Dressing

Preparation Time: 5 Minutes

Cooking Time: 0 Minutes

Servings: 2

Ingredients:

- 3 tablespoons honey
- 1 teaspoon Dijon mustard
- ¼ teaspoon sesame oil
- 1 pinch red pepper flakes
- 1½ tablespoons rice wine vinegar
- ¼ cup mayonnaise
- Salt and pepper to taste

Directions:

1. In a small bowl, mix all ingredients together. Then, refrigerate. Serve on salads.

Nutrition: Calories: 322; Total Fat: 16.4g; Saturated Fat: 9.3g; Protein: 3.1g; Carbs: 43.6g; Fiber: 1.9g; Sugar: 32.6g

El Charro Café's Hot Chocolate

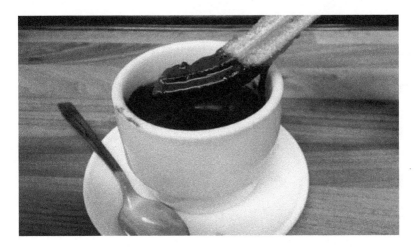

Preparation Time: 5 Minutes

Cooking Time: 10 Minutes

Servings: 4

Ingredients:

- 6 cups whole milk
- 1 cup sugar
- 6 tablespoons cocoa powder or 4 squares Ibarra Mexican chocolate
- 1 teaspoon ground cinnamon
- 1 teaspoon vanilla extract

Directions:

1. Combine all the ingredients in a saucepan.
2. Warm over medium heat, stirring constantly. Do not boil the mixture.

3. Remove from heat. Then, use a hand whisk to whisk until frothy.

4. Pour chocolate into mugs and serve.

Nutrition: Calories: 580; Total Fat: 21.8g; Saturated Fat: 11.8g; Protein: 9.1g; Carbs: 88.5g; Fiber: 3.4g; Sugar: 32.6g

Chi Chi's Bloody Mary

Preparation Time: 5 Minutes

Cooking Time: 0 Minutes

Servings: 2

Ingredients:

- 1 cup thick chunky salsa, medium
- ¼ cup vodka
- 1 teaspoon lemon juice
- 1 teaspoon Worcestershire sauce
- ¼ teaspoon hot pepper sauce
- 4–6 olives
- 2–3 celery sticks

Directions:

1. Blend all the ingredients in a blender until smooth.
2. Pour into an ice-filled cocktail shaker and shake well.
3. Strain into glasses and add more ice.
4. Garnish with olives and celery, if desired.

Nutrition: Calories: 358; Total Fat: 19.5g; Saturated Fat: 3g; Protein: 3.9g; Carbs: 46.8g; Fiber: 1.6g; Sugar: 24.3g

Spinach Artichoke Dip

Preparation Time: 5 Minutes

Cooking Time: 10 Minutes

Servings: 8

Ingredients:

- 3 tablespoons butter
- 3 tablespoons flour
- 1½ cups milk
- ½ teaspoon salt
- ¼ teaspoon black pepper
- 5 ounces spinach, frozen and chopped
- ¼ cup artichokes, diced
- ½ teaspoon chopped garlic
- ½ cup parmesan, shredded
- ½ cup mozzarella, shredded
- 1 tablespoon asiago cheese, shredded
- 1 tablespoon Romano cheese, shredded
- 2 tablespoons cream cheese
- ¼ cup mozzarella cheese, for topping

Directions:

1. First, melt butter over medium heat in a saucepan.

2. Add flour and cook for about 1–2 minutes. Add milk and stir until thick.

3. Season with salt and pepper to taste. Add spinach, diced artichokes, garlic, cheeses and cream cheese to the pan. Stir until warmed.

4. Lastly, pour into a small baking dish. Sprinkle mozzarella cheese on top. Then, place under the broiler. Broil until the top begins browning.

Nutrition: Calories: 415; Total Fat: 25.8g; Saturated Fat: 7.9g; Protein: 4.8g; Carbs: 44g; Fiber: 1.8g; Sugar: 28.9g

New York Cheesecake

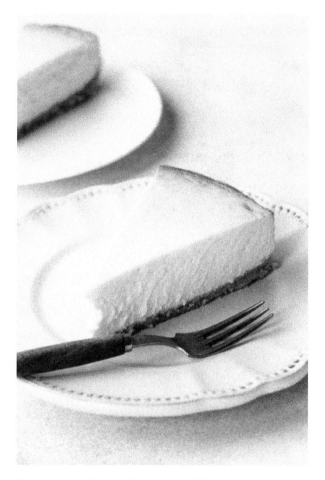

Preparation Time: 5 Minutes

Cooking Time: 55 Minutes

Servings: 12

Ingredients:

- 5 (approximately 8 ounces) packages cream cheese, softened

- 1¾ cups sugar
- 2 cups graham cracker crumbs, finely crushed
- ½ cup butter or ½ cup margarine, melted
- 2 large egg yolks
- 1½ teaspoons vanilla
- 5 large eggs
- 1 teaspoon lemon, finely shredded
- 2 tablespoons all-purpose flour
- 1/3 cup whipping cream

Directions:

1. Combine the graham cracker crumbs with melted butter in a bowl; give it a good stir until combined well.

2. Press onto the bottom & approximately 2 ½ inches up the sides of a 9x3-inch spring-form pan. Combine the cream cheese with flour, vanilla & sugar; mix well. Beat using an electric mixer, on low speed until fluffy.

3. Add egg yolks and eggs; continue to beat until just combined, on low speed. Stir in the lemon peel and whipping cream. Pour into the prepared pan. Place pan in a shallow baking pan in the oven.

4. Bake until the middle appears nearly set, for 1 ½ hours, at 325 F. Let cool for 10 to 15 minutes. Loosen the crust from sides of pan.

5. Cool for half an hour more and then remove sides of pan. Let completely cool and then chill for overnight.

6. Just before serving, don't forget to garnish your cake with some fresh berries.

Nutrition: Calories: 732; Total Fat: 47.6g; Saturated Fat: 18.1g; Protein: 26.9g; Carbs: 48.9g; Fiber: 4.3g; Sugar: 7.4g

Carrabba's Dessert Rosa

Preparation Time: 5 Minutes

Cooking Time: 45 Minutes

Servings: 12

Ingredients:

- 1 box white cake mix
- 1 butter stick
- 6 egg yolks
- ½ cup sugar, divided
- 4 tablespoons all-purpose flour
- 1 pinch salt
- 2 cups milk
- 3 teaspoons vanilla extract, divided
- 8 strawberries, sliced
- 2 bananas, sliced
- 1 can crushed pineapple
- 1 cup heavy cream
- ¼ cup sugar
- Chocolate syrup

Directions:

1. Make cake according to the package instructions but replace oil with butter. Then, set aside to cool.

2. Start making pastry cream by adding egg yolks and ¼ cup sugar to a bowl. Mix until smooth and liquid becomes lighter in color. Stir in flour and salt until combined. Set aside.

3. Heat milk, remaining sugar and 2 teaspoons vanilla extract in a saucepan over medium heat and boil. Then, while stirring, gradually pour about half of scalding milk mixture into egg yolk/sugar mixture. Return saucepan to heat and pour in egg yolk/sugar mixture. Continue to stir until sauce comes to a boil Continue boiling for about 1 minute or until cream thickens, stirring continuously. Turn off heat, then pour into a bowl. Mix in butter until melted. Cover with bowl with plastic wrap and refrigerate for 1 hour.

4. For the fruit topping, add strawberries and bananas into individual bowls, unmixed, and pour in juice of canned pineapples. Add pineapples to a separate bowl. For whipped

cream, whisk heavy cream in a bowl until a bit firm. Whisk in sugar and remaining vanilla extract until you can form a firm peak.

5. Assemble cake by slicing it into two layers. Return 1st layer onto pan, then layer with pineapple and pastry cream. Top with 2nd cake layer, then top with strawberries, followed by bananas. Drizzle chocolate syrup on top.

6. Right before serving, spread whipped cream onto individual cake slices.

Nutrition: Calories: 448; Total Fat: 30.1g; Saturated Fat: 14.7g; Protein: 27.8g; Carbs: 17.4g; Fiber: 1.9g; Sugar: 4.8g

Starbucks' Iced Lemon Pound Cake

Preparation Time: 5 Minutes

Cooking Time: 50 Minutes

Servings: 8

Ingredients:

Loaf

- 1½ cups all-purpose flour
- ½ teaspoon salt
- 2 teaspoons baking powder
- 3 large eggs
- 1 cup sour cream
- 1 cup granulated sugar
- ½ cup vegetable oil
- 2 tablespoons lemon zest
- 1 tablespoon lemon extract, or to taste

Lemon Glaze

- 3 tablespoons lemon juice
- 1 cup powdered sugar

Directions:

1. Preheat oven to 350°F. Grease and flour a loaf pan.

2. Next, in a bowl, combine baking powder, flour and salt. Set aside.

3. In a mixer bowl, beat the eggs, sugar and sour cream until well-blended.

4. Continue beating while adding oil in a stream.

5. Add lemon zest and extract and mix.

6. Next, add the flour mixture. Mix just to incorporate. The batter will be lumpy.

7. Pour batter into prepared loaf pan and spread evenly with a spatula.

8. Then, bake for 40 minutes and then tent with foil.

9. Let bake until toothpick inserted at the center comes out with just a few crumbs (about 10–12 minutes).

10.   Place pan on a wire rack for loaf to cool completely.

11.   Meanwhile, prepare the glaze. Whisk powdered sugar while adding lemon juice gradually until the right consistency is achieved.

12.   Lastly, remove loaf from pan and drizzle with glaze.

Nutrition: Calories: 674; Total Fat: 49.1g; Saturated Fat: 23.4g; Protein: 13.3g; Carbs: 46.1g; Fiber: 3.8g; Sugar: 2.5g

Buca Di Beppo's Tiramisu

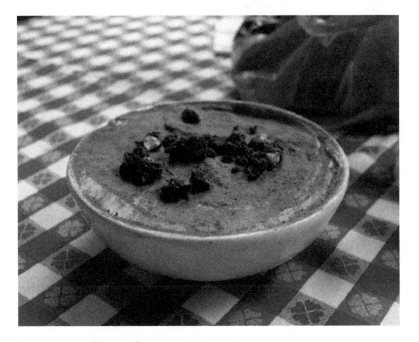

Preparation Time: 5 Minutes

Cooking Time: 0 Minutes

Servings: 2

Ingredients:

- 3 6-inch pieces round savoiardi
- ½ cup espresso rum mix
- 3 ounces zabaglione custard
- 9 ounces sweet mascarpone
- ½ ounce cocoa powder
- 1/8 cup biscotti, crumbled

Directions:

1. Dip one round savoiardi in espresso rum mix and place in serving bowl (about 3 inches deep and 7 inches wide).
2. Spread with a third of the zabaglione, then a third of the mascarpone.
3. Repeat with the rest of the dipped biscuits, zabaglione and mascarpone, to make 3 layers.
4. Chill before serving.
5. Sprinkle with cocoa powder and crumbled biscotti.

Nutrition: Calories: 197; Total Fat: 9g; Saturated Fat: 2.8g; Protein: 3.9g; Carbs: 24.8g; Fiber: 0.8g; Sugar: 1.1g

CONCLUSION

Thank you for downloading this book, "Copycat Recipes Cookbook".

I hope that you will find the recipes in this cookbook useful, and that they will help you to create delicious and healthful meals for your family.

Copycat recipes are very popular because they are cheap, delicious and you can cook them for the family in a short time.

For those who don't know what a "copycat" is, let me explain. Copycat recipes are homemade versions of the meals served in restaurants. It's a good idea to learn how to cook them at home, so that you can save money on dining out, and enjoy restaurant-quality food instead of fast food or frozen dinners.

My goal is to provide you with lots of delicious, easy copycat recipes. I know that you'll love these recipes and that they will become family favorites.

The recipes in this book were collected from various sources on the Internet, like blogs and forums, however all of them have been thoroughly tested before being added to the book.

This cookbook contains a collection of recipes that are similar, in some way, to familiar dishes. The intent behind this cookbook is to create alternates to the original dishes that may be more appropriate for people who need or prefer a lower-salt diet.

Here are things to remember when you are cooking:

1. When you are cooking a recipe, always follow the instructions as written. If the instruction calls for 4 Tbsp of butter, use 4 Tbsp of butter. However, there are some ingredients that you can reduce or substitute if you don't like a certain ingredient and/or if you wish to reduce the salt content.

2. Feel free to substitute your favorite spices in place of a spice called for in a recipe: however, be aware of the volume and/or weight of spices when making substitutions since some spices

are stronger than others and can result in an overly-spiced dish.

3. Use the recipes as written, and be sure to note any substitutions you have made.

4. You may choose to share your family's favorite recipes with others on social media.

5. When cooking, you may wish to occasionally monitor the times, temperatures, and/or quantities as it is difficult to always remember all the ways that a recipe has been adjusted.

6. Some of the recipes call for fresh herbs. If you don't have them, you can use dried herbs instead; but keep in mind that dried herbs are more concentrated and often stronger than fresh, so use less.

I hope that you enjoy this cookbook and that it will inspire you to cook for your family.

- PS, this is a really simple diet book. If you are looking for the "super-secret" or the "secret ingredient" to a diet, don't look here. This is a very simple book with some basic nutrition information and some basic recommendations about what's good for you in terms of food choices.

If you do cook from this book, I'd be really glad to hear about it.

Good luck in your cooking!

CPSIA information can be obtained
at www.ICGtesting.com
Printed in the USA
BVHW011431140421
604747BV00028B/315